Chair Yoga for Seniors To Lose Weight

28 Days challenge to Elevate Your Well-Being with 10-Minute Step-by-Step Exercises for Weight Loss and Flexibility Over 60

Property of

Eleanor Grace

Intentionally left blank

Copyright Notice

Disclaimer:

The information provided in "Chair Yoga for Senior Weight Loss" is intended for general informational purposes only. The author, Eleanor Grace, is not a medical professional, and the content should not be construed as medical advice, diagnosis, or treatment. Always consult with a qualified healthcare provider for advice regarding medical conditions or concerns. Reliance on any information provided in this guide is at your own risk.

Legal Notice:

DEDICATION

To the resilient, the wise, and the ageless in spirit,

This guide is lovingly offered to every senior embracing the practice of chair yoga. It is not merely a physical exercise but a celebration of the beauty that accompanies the passing years.

Your unwavering determination, the laughter lines that tell stories of a lifetime, and the depth of your experiences have inspired the creation of this guide.

In honor of those who have gracefully navigated life's journey, may these chair yoga exercises become a source of strength, joy, and a reminder that vitality knows no bounds.

With deepest respect and admiration,

This guide is dedicated to you.

May each stretch, each breath, and every moment spent within these pages be a tribute to the remarkable tapestry of your lives.

Here's to the elders, the mentors, the grandparents, and all those who continue to illuminate the world with their wisdom, laughter, and enduring spirit.

With gratitude and admiration,

Eleanor Grace

Table of Contents

Chapter 1: Introduction to Chair Yoga for Weight Loss

Are you ready to embark on a transformative journey towards better health and well-being? Picture this: Imagine waking up every morning feeling energized, vibrant, and full of vitality. Envision moving through your day with ease and grace, free from the limitations of stiffness and discomfort. Close your eyes and visualize yourself achieving your weight loss goals, not through grueling workouts or restrictive diets, but through the gentle, accessible practice of chair yoga.

As a seasoned yoga coach with a passion for empowering seniors to live their best lives, I've witnessed firsthand the remarkable impact that chair yoga can have on physical fitness, mental clarity, and emotional balance. Through years of dedicated practice and teaching, I've seen countless individuals experience profound transformations in their bodies and minds, simply by incorporating chair yoga into their daily routines.

But perhaps you're skeptical. You might be thinking, "Can yoga really help me lose weight?" The answer is a resounding yes! Chair yoga may not involve intense cardio sessions or heavy lifting, but it offers a holistic approach to weight loss that addresses the body, mind, and spirit. By engaging in gentle yet effective movements, deep breathing exercises, and mindful meditation, you can awaken your body's natural ability to shed excess pounds and find balance from within.

Consider the story of Margaret, a vibrant woman in her 70s who struggled with arthritis and mobility issues. Frustrated by her limited range of motion and lack of energy, Margaret was hesitant to try chair yoga at first. However, with gentle encouragement and support, she decided to give it a chance. Within just a few weeks of consistent practice, Margaret noticed significant improvements in her flexibility, strength, and overall well-being. Not only did she experience relief from her arthritis symptoms, but she also began to shed unwanted pounds and regain her confidence in her body's abilities.

Then there's David, a retiree who had battled with weight gain and high blood pressure for years. Tired of relying on medication to manage his health issues, David was determined to make a change. Through a tailored chair yoga program focused on cardiovascular health and stress reduction, David not only lost weight but also saw a dramatic improvement in his blood pressure readings. He credits chair yoga with not only transforming his physical health but also instilling a sense of inner peace and resilience that he had never experienced before.

These stories are just a glimpse of the countless success stories that unfold every day on the mat. Whether you're a senior looking to lose weight, improve flexibility, or simply enhance your overall quality of life, chair yoga offers a safe, accessible, and enjoyable path to wellness. In the pages that follow, you'll discover a wealth of practical tips, step-by-step exercises, and expert guidance to help you unlock the full potential of chair yoga and embark on your own journey towards optimal health and vitality.

So, are you ready to take the first step towards a healthier, happier you? Let's roll out our mats, take a deep breath, and begin this transformative adventure together. Your body, mind, and spirit will thank you for it. Welcome to Chair Yoga for Senior Weight Loss—a journey of self-discovery, empowerment, and infinite possibilities.

Understanding Chair Yoga and Its Benefits for Seniors

Chair yoga is more than just a series of gentle movements; it's a gateway to holistic wellness that can transform the lives of seniors in profound ways. Unlike traditional yoga, which often involves complex poses and challenging sequences, chair yoga offers a modified approach that is accessible to individuals of all ages and fitness levels. By adapting traditional yoga poses to be performed while seated or using a chair for support, chair yoga provides a safe and effective way for seniors to improve their strength, flexibility, and overall well-being.

As a yoga coach with years of experience working with seniors, I've witnessed firsthand the remarkable benefits that chair yoga can offer. From easing joint pain and stiffness to improving balance and mental clarity, the positive effects of chair yoga extend far beyond the physical realm. By incorporating gentle stretches, controlled breathing techniques, and mindful meditation practices, seniors can cultivate a deeper sense of connection to their bodies and minds, fostering a greater sense of peace and tranquility in their daily lives.

One of the key advantages of chair yoga is its adaptability to individual needs and abilities. Whether you're recovering from an injury, managing a chronic condition, or simply looking to stay active as you age, chair yoga can be tailored to suit your unique circumstances. By using props such as chairs, bolsters, and blocks, you can modify poses to accommodate limitations in mobility or flexibility, ensuring a safe and comfortable practice that honors your body's needs.

Importance of Safe and Effective Exercise for Weight Loss

When it comes to weight loss, the old adage "slow and steady wins the race" couldn't be more true, especially for seniors. While crash diets and extreme exercise regimens may promise quick results, they often lead to unsustainable outcomes and can even jeopardize your health in the long run. That's where chair yoga comes in. By providing a low-impact, gentle form of exercise that can be easily integrated into your daily routine, chair yoga offers a safe and effective approach to weight loss that focuses on sustainable, long-term results.

As someone who has struggled with weight management in the past, I understand the challenges that seniors face when it comes to losing weight. It's not just about shedding pounds; it's about cultivating a healthy relationship with food and exercise, nurturing your body from the inside out. Chair yoga offers a holistic solution that addresses both the physical and emotional aspects of weight loss, helping you to build strength, confidence, and resilience along the way.

● ● ●

Setting Realistic Goals for Senior Weight Loss Journey

Setting realistic goals is essential for success on any weight loss journey, especially for seniors. Rather than focusing solely on the number on the scale, consider setting goals that are centered around improving your overall health and well-being. Whether it's increasing your daily activity level, incorporating more whole foods into your diet, or simply finding moments of joy and gratitude in each day, small, achievable goals can add up to significant progress over time.

When setting goals for your chair yoga practice, it's important to take into account your current level of fitness and any physical limitations you may have. Start by identifying areas where you'd like to see improvement, whether it's increasing flexibility, building strength, or reducing stress. Then, break down your goals into manageable steps, setting realistic milestones along the way. By celebrating each small victory, you'll stay motivated and inspired to continue on your journey towards optimal health and vitality.

In conclusion, chair yoga offers seniors a gentle yet powerful tool for achieving their weight loss goals in a safe and sustainable manner. By understanding the benefits of chair yoga, prioritizing safe and effective exercise practices, and setting realistic goals for your journey, you can unlock the full potential of this transformative practice and embark on a path towards a healthier, happier you.

WHY CHAIR YOGA ?

Chair yoga offers a myriad of benefits that make it an ideal choice for seniors seeking to improve their health and well-being. Here's why chair yoga is such a valuable practice:

Accessibility: Chair yoga is accessible to individuals of all ages and fitness levels, making it an inclusive option for seniors who may have mobility issues, balance concerns, or other physical limitations. By utilizing a chair for support, participants can comfortably perform a wide range of yoga poses without the need to get down on the floor, ensuring a safe and enjoyable practice for everyone.

Gentleness: Chair yoga focuses on gentle movements and stretches that are easy on the joints and muscles, making it ideal for seniors who may be dealing with conditions like arthritis, osteoporosis, or chronic pain. The controlled, low-impact nature of chair yoga helps to reduce the risk of injury while still providing significant benefits for strength, flexibility, and mobility.

Improves Flexibility and Mobility: Despite being performed in a seated position, chair yoga is highly effective at improving flexibility and mobility throughout the body. By gently stretching and lengthening muscles, tendons, and ligaments, chair yoga helps to increase range of motion, alleviate stiffness, and enhance overall mobility, making everyday activities easier and more comfortable.

Strengthens Muscles: Chair yoga incorporates a variety of resistance-based exercises that target major muscle groups, helping to build strength and stability throughout the body. From chair squats to seated leg lifts, these strengthening poses help seniors maintain muscle mass, improve balance, and reduce the risk of falls, which is particularly important as we age.

Promotes Relaxation and Stress Reduction: Chair yoga incorporates deep breathing techniques, relaxation exercises, and mindfulness practices that promote a sense of calm and tranquility. By focusing on the breath and cultivating present-moment awareness, seniors can reduce stress levels, lower blood pressure, and improve overall mental well-being, leading to greater resilience and emotional balance.

Enhances Mental Clarity and Focus: Chair yoga encourages participants to cultivate mindfulness and concentration, which can have profound effects on cognitive function and mental clarity. By practicing present-moment awareness and focusing on the sensations of the body, seniors can sharpen their cognitive skills, enhance memory, and boost overall brain health.

Encourages Social Connection: Chair yoga classes provide an opportunity for seniors to connect with others in a supportive and nurturing environment. By participating in group sessions, seniors can share experiences, exchange encouragement, and build meaningful connections with like-minded individuals, fostering a sense of belonging and community.

Overall, chair yoga offers seniors a gentle yet powerful pathway to improved health, vitality, and quality of life. Whether you're looking to increase flexibility, build strength, reduce stress, or simply enjoy the benefits of a mindful movement practice, chair yoga provides a safe, accessible, and enjoyable option for seniors of all abilities.

Chapter 2: Getting Your Equipment Ready

Embarking on your chair yoga journey requires some essential equipment to ensure a safe and comfortable practice experience. In this chapter, we'll explore the necessary gear, offer tips for selecting the right chair and accessories, and discuss how to create a supportive environment for your chair yoga workouts.

Essential Equipment for Chair Yoga Practice for Seniors

1. Chair: The cornerstone of chair yoga practice, your chair should be sturdy, stable, and without wheels. Opt for a chair with a straight back and no armrests to allow for a full range of motion during poses. Ensure that the seat is comfortable and at a height that allows your feet to rest flat on the floor.

2. Yoga Mat: While not strictly necessary for chair yoga, a yoga mat can provide added cushioning and stability, especially if your chair has a slippery surface. Choose a non-slip mat that is thick enough to cushion your joints but not too thick that it interferes with your stability on the chair.

3. Props: Depending on your needs and preferences, you may want to have some props on hand to enhance your practice. Common props for chair yoga include yoga blocks, yoga straps, and bolsters. These props can help you modify poses, deepen stretches, and provide additional support where needed.

4. Comfortable Clothing: Wear loose, breathable clothing that allows for freedom of movement. Avoid clothing with tight waistbands or restrictive seams that could dig into your skin during practice. Opt for layers that you can easily remove or adjust as needed to maintain a comfortable body temperature.

Tips for Choosing the Right Chair and Accessories

1. Chair Height: When selecting a chair for chair yoga practice, ensure that it is at a height that allows your feet to rest comfortably flat on the floor. If necessary, you can adjust the height of your chair by placing cushions or yoga blocks underneath.

2. Chair Stability: Choose a chair that is stable and secure, with sturdy legs that can support your weight without wobbling or tipping over. Avoid chairs with wheels or swivel bases, as these can make it difficult to maintain proper alignment during practice.

3. Chair Material: Look for a chair with a smooth, flat surface that provides a comfortable base for sitting and moving. Avoid chairs with cushions or padding that are too soft, as they may not provide enough support for certain poses.

4. Accessories: Consider investing in accessories such as non-slip pads or grip socks to enhance the stability of your chair and prevent it from sliding on smooth surfaces. Additionally, you may want to have a water bottle and towel nearby to stay hydrated and wipe away any sweat during your practice.

Creating a Safe and Supportive Environment for Chair Yoga Workouts

1. Clear Space: Choose a quiet, clutter-free area with enough room to move freely around your chair. Ensure that there are no obstacles or hazards that could cause you to trip or fall during practice.

2. Good Lighting: Make sure the space is well-lit with natural or artificial light so that you can see clearly and avoid straining your eyes during practice. Consider using soft, diffused lighting to create a calming ambiance.

3. Comfortable Temperature: Maintain a comfortable temperature in the practice space to prevent overheating or feeling too cold during your workout. Dress in layers so that you can adjust your clothing as needed to stay comfortable.

4. Supportive Atmosphere: Create a supportive atmosphere for your chair yoga practice by playing soft music, lighting candles, or incorporating aromatherapy scents that promote relaxation and focus. Surround yourself with objects that inspire and uplift you, such as photos, plants, or inspirational quotes.

By taking the time to gather the necessary equipment, choose the right chair and accessories, and create a safe and supportive environment for your chair yoga workouts, you'll set yourself up for success in your practice journey. Remember, the most important thing is to listen to your body and honor its needs throughout your practice. With dedication, patience, and a little bit of preparation, you'll soon be reaping the countless benefits of chair yoga.

Chapter 3: Simple Chair Yoga Poses for Daily Practice

In this chapter, we'll explore four simple yet effective chair yoga poses that you can incorporate into your daily routine. These poses are gentle, accessible, and designed to promote flexibility, mobility, and relaxation. Below, you'll find step-by-step instructions for each pose, along with their benefits and recommended durations.

1. Seated Cat-Cow Stretch

Steps:

- Sit comfortably on your chair with your feet flat on the floor and your hands resting on your thighs.

- Inhale as you arch your spine, lifting your chest and tilting your pelvis forward (Cow Pose).

- Exhale as you round your spine, tucking your chin to your chest and drawing your belly button towards your spine (Cat Pose).

- Continue to flow smoothly between Cat and Cow Poses, coordinating your breath with your movement.

Benefits:

- Improves spinal flexibility and mobility.

- Releases tension in the back, neck, and shoulders.

- Stimulates digestion and massages the internal organs.

- Promotes relaxation and stress relief.

Duration: Repeat the Cat-Cow stretch for 5-10 breaths, flowing gently with each inhale and exhale.

2. Seated Forward Fold

Steps:

- Sit tall on your chair with your feet hip-width apart and your hands resting on your thighs.

- Inhale deeply, lengthening your spine and lifting your chest towards the sky.

- Exhale as you hinge forward from your hips, reaching your hands towards your feet or the floor.

- Allow your head to hang heavy and relax your neck and shoulders.

- Hold the forward fold for several breaths, feeling a gentle stretch along the back of your legs and spine.

Benefits:

- Stretches the spine, hamstrings, and lower back.

- Relieves tension in the neck and shoulders.

- Calms the mind and promotes relaxation.

- Stimulates the digestive system and improves circulation.

Duration: Hold the seated forward fold for 30-60 seconds, breathing deeply and surrendering to the stretch.

3. Seated Spinal Twist

Steps:

- Sit sideways on your chair with your feet flat on the floor and your spine tall.

- Inhale to lengthen your spine, then exhale as you twist your torso towards the back of the chair, placing one hand on the backrest for support and the other hand on your opposite knee.

- Gently deepen the twist with each exhale, using your breath to guide you deeper into the pose.

- Keep your shoulders relaxed and your gaze soft, avoiding any strain or discomfort in your neck or spine.

Benefits:

- Improves spinal mobility and flexibility.

- Stretches the muscles along the spine, shoulders, and chest.

- Stimulates digestion and massages the internal organs.

- Releases tension and promotes relaxation.

Duration: Hold the seated spinal twist for 5-10 breaths on each side, focusing on maintaining length in the spine and openness in the chest.

4. Seated Side Stretch

Steps:

- Sit tall on your chair with your feet flat on the floor and your hands resting on your thighs.

- Inhale deeply, lengthening your spine and reaching your arms overhead.

- Exhale as you lean gently to one side, keeping both hips rooted firmly in the chair.

- Reach through your fingertips and feel a stretch along the side of your body, from your fingertips to your hip.

- Hold the stretch for several breaths, then inhale to return to center and repeat on the other side.

Benefits:

- Stretches the muscles along the sides of the torso and waist.

- Opens up the chest and improves lung capacity.

- Increases flexibility in the spine and shoulders.

- Promotes relaxation and mental clarity.

Duration: Hold the seated side stretch for 30-60 seconds on each side, breathing deeply and surrendering to the stretch.

5. Seated Neck Stretch

Steps:

1. Sit comfortably on your chair with your feet flat on the floor and your spine tall.

2. Inhale deeply and lengthen your spine, feeling a gentle lift through the crown of your head.

3. Exhale as you tilt your head to one side, bringing your ear towards your shoulder.

4. Use your hand to gently press down on the opposite side of your head, increasing the stretch along the side of your neck.

5. Hold the stretch for several breaths, then inhale to return to center and repeat on the other side.

Benefits:

- Relieves tension and stiffness in the neck muscles.

- Improves range of motion in the neck and shoulders.

- Alleviates headaches and neck pain.

- Promotes relaxation and stress relief.

Duration: Hold the seated neck stretch for 20-30 seconds on each side, breathing deeply and allowing the tension to melt away.

6. Seated Shoulder Rolls

Steps:

1. Sit tall on your chair with your feet flat on the floor and your hands resting on your thighs.

2. Inhale deeply and lift your shoulders up towards your ears, creating tension in the shoulder muscles.

3. Exhale as you roll your shoulders back and down, drawing big circles with your shoulders.

4. Continue to flow smoothly through the shoulder rolls, coordinating your breath with your movement.

5. After several repetitions, reverse the direction of the shoulder rolls, moving them forward instead of backward.

Benefits:

- Releases tension and tightness in the shoulders and upper back.

- Improves circulation and blood flow to the shoulder muscles.

- Increases shoulder mobility and range of motion.

- Promotes relaxation and reduces stress.

Duration: Perform 10-15 seated shoulder rolls in each direction, focusing on maintaining smooth, controlled movements and deep breathing throughout.

7. Seated Hip Opener

Steps:

1. Sit comfortably on your chair with your feet flat on the floor and your spine tall.

2. Place your hands on your knees and inhale deeply, lengthening your spine.

3. Exhale as you gently press one knee out to the side, opening up your hip.

4. Hold the stretch for a few breaths, feeling a gentle opening in the hip joint.

5. Inhale to return to center, then repeat on the other side.

Benefits:

- Increases flexibility and mobility in the hip joints.

- Relieves tension and tightness in the hips and groin.

- Improves posture and alignment.

- Stimulates circulation and blood flow to the hip muscles.

Duration: Hold the seated hip opener for 20-30 seconds on each side, breathing deeply and focusing on relaxing into the stretch.

8. Seated Knee to Chest Stretch

Steps:

1. Sit tall on your chair with your feet flat on the floor and your hands resting on your thighs.

2. Inhale deeply and lift one knee towards your chest, hugging it in with both hands.

3. Exhale as you gently press the knee towards your chest, feeling a stretch in the hip and lower back.

4. Hold the stretch for a few breaths, then release and repeat on the other side.

5. For a deeper stretch, you can gently rock the knee from side to side or in small circles.

Benefits:

- Stretches the muscles of the lower back, hips, and glutes.

- Relieves tension and tightness in the lower body.

- Improves flexibility and range of motion in the hip joints.

- Promotes relaxation and stress relief.

Duration: Hold the seated knee to chest stretch for 20-30 seconds on each side, breathing deeply and allowing the muscles to soften and release.

9. Seated Ankle Circles

Steps:

1. Sit comfortably on your chair with your feet flat on the floor.

2. Lift one foot off the ground and begin to rotate your ankle in a circular motion.

3. Start with small circles and gradually increase the size as you warm up the ankle joint.

4. After several rotations in one direction, switch to the other direction.

5. Repeat the ankle circles with the other foot.

Benefits:

- Increases mobility and flexibility in the ankles.

- Helps to reduce stiffness and improve circulation in the feet and lower legs.

- Can relieve tension and discomfort caused by prolonged sitting or standing.

- Promotes better balance and stability.

Duration: Perform 10-15 ankle circles in each direction with each foot, focusing on smooth, controlled movements.

10. Seated Heart Opener

Steps:

1. Sit tall on your chair with your feet flat on the floor and your hands resting on your thighs.

2. Inhale deeply as you lift your chest towards the sky, arching your upper back slightly.

3. Draw your shoulder blades down and back, opening up the front of your chest.

4. Allow your head to tilt back slightly if it feels comfortable, but avoid straining your neck.

5. Hold the heart opener for several breaths, feeling a gentle stretch across the front of your chest.

Benefits:

- Improves posture and counteracts the effects of hunching over.

- Opens up the chest and lungs, promoting better breathing.

- Releases tension in the shoulders and upper back.

- Invokes feelings of openness, vulnerability, and emotional release.

Duration: Hold the seated heart opener for 30-60 seconds, breathing deeply and surrendering to the stretch.

11. Seated Gentle Twist

Steps:

1. Sit sideways on your chair with your feet flat on the floor and your spine tall.

2. Inhale deeply as you lengthen your spine, then exhale as you twist your torso towards the back of the chair.

3. Place one hand on the backrest for support and the other hand on your opposite knee.

4. Gently deepen the twist with each exhale, using your breath to guide you deeper into the pose.

5. Keep your shoulders relaxed and your gaze soft, avoiding any strain or discomfort in your neck or spine.

6. Hold the twist for several breaths, then inhale to return to center and repeat on the other side.

Benefits:

- Improves spinal mobility and flexibility.

- Stimulates digestion and massages the internal organs.

- Relieves tension in the back, shoulders, and neck.

- Promotes detoxification and elimination of waste from the body.

Duration: Hold the seated gentle twist for 5-10 breaths on each side, focusing on maintaining length in the spine and openness in the chest.

12. Seated Side Bends

Steps:

1. Sit tall on your chair with your feet flat on the floor and your hands resting on your thighs.

2. Inhale deeply as you lengthen your spine, then exhale as you gently lean to one side, bringing your ear towards your shoulder.

3. Keep both hips rooted firmly in the chair and avoid collapsing into the side bend.

4. Reach through your fingertips and feel a stretch along the side of your body, from your fingertips to your hip.

5. Hold the stretch for several breaths, then inhale to return to center and repeat on the other side.

Benefits:

- Stretches the muscles along the sides of the torso and waist.

- Opens up the chest and improves lung capacity.

- Increases flexibility in the spine and shoulders.

- Promotes relaxation and mental clarity.

Duration: Hold the seated side bend for 30-60 seconds on each side, breathing deeply and surrendering to the stretch.

13. Seated Chest Opener

Steps:

1. Sit comfortably on your chair with your feet flat on the floor and your spine tall.

2. Interlace your fingers behind your back, palms facing each other.

3. Inhale deeply as you squeeze your shoulder blades together and lift your chest towards the ceiling.

4. Keep your chin parallel to the floor and your gaze forward.

5. Hold the stretch for several breaths, feeling a gentle opening in the chest and shoulders.

6. Exhale to release the stretch and return to the starting position.

Benefits:

- Opens up the chest and shoulders.

- Improves posture by counteracting the effects of slouching.

- Releases tension and tightness in the upper body.

- Stimulates deep breathing and enhances lung capacity.

Duration: Hold the seated chest opener for 30-60 seconds, breathing deeply and consciously expanding your chest with each inhale.

14. Seated Wrist Stretches

Steps:

1. Sit tall on your chair with your feet flat on the floor and your arms extended in front of you.

2. Extend your right arm forward with your palm facing down.

3. Use your left hand to gently press down on the fingers of your right hand, stretching the wrist and forearm.

4. Hold the stretch for a few breaths, feeling a gentle stretch along the underside of your wrist.

5. Release the stretch and switch sides, repeating with your left hand.

6. Alternatively, you can perform wrist circles by rotating your wrists in a circular motion, first clockwise and then counterclockwise.

Benefits:

- Relieves tension and stiffness in the wrists and forearms.

- Improves flexibility and range of motion in the wrists.

- Alleviates symptoms of carpal tunnel syndrome and repetitive strain injuries.

- Promotes circulation and reduces swelling in the hands and fingers.

Duration: Hold each wrist stretch for 15-30 seconds on each side, repeating as needed to release tension and increase flexibility.

15. Seated Leg Extensions

Steps:

1. Sit tall on your chair with your feet flat on the floor and your hands resting on your thighs.

2. Extend your right leg forward, keeping your knee straight and your foot flexed.

3. Hold the position for a few breaths, feeling a gentle stretch along the back of your leg.

4. Flex and point your toes a few times to release tension in the calf muscles.

5. Lower your right leg and repeat the stretch with your left leg.

6. For a deeper stretch, you can gently hinge forward from your hips while keeping your back straight.

Benefits:

- Stretches the hamstrings and calf muscles.

- Improves flexibility and range of motion in the legs.

- Enhances circulation and reduces stiffness in the lower body.

- Helps to alleviate symptoms of sciatica and lower back pain.

Duration: Hold each leg extension for 15-30 seconds, breathing deeply and surrendering to the stretch.

16. Seated Butterfly Stretch

Steps:

1. Sit tall on your chair with your feet flat on the floor and your knees bent.

2. Bring the soles of your feet together, allowing your knees to open out to the sides.

3. Hold onto your ankles or feet with your hands, gently pressing down on your thighs to deepen the stretch.

4. Sit up tall and lengthen through your spine, avoiding rounding or collapsing in the upper body.

5. Hold the stretch for several breaths, feeling a gentle opening in the hips and groin.

6. To increase the stretch, you can gently press your elbows into your inner thighs while keeping your spine long.

Benefits:

- Opens up the hips and groin.

- Stretches the inner thighs and groin muscles.

- Improves flexibility and range of motion in the hips.

- Relieves tension and stiffness in the lower body.

Duration: Hold the seated butterfly stretch for 30-60 seconds, breathing deeply and allowing the hips to relax and open with each breath.

17. Seated Hamstring Stretch

Steps:

- Sit comfortably on the edge of your chair with your feet flat on the floor and your knees bent.

- Extend one leg out in front of you, keeping the foot flexed and the heel on the ground.

- Inhale deeply to lengthen your spine, then exhale as you hinge forward from your hips, reaching towards your extended foot.

- Keep your back straight and your chest lifted, avoiding any rounding of the spine.

- Hold the stretch for several breaths, feeling a gentle stretch along the back of your extended leg.

- Repeat on the other side.

Benefits:

- Stretches the hamstrings, improving flexibility and mobility in the back of the legs.

- Relieves tension in the lower back and hips.

- Stimulates circulation and promotes relaxation.

Duration: Hold the seated hamstring stretch for 30-60 seconds on each leg, breathing deeply and surrendering to the stretch.

18. Seated Calf Stretch

Steps:

- Sit tall on your chair with your feet flat on the floor and your knees bent at a 90-degree angle.

- Extend one leg out in front of you, keeping the foot flexed and the toes pointing towards the ceiling.

- Inhale deeply to lengthen your spine, then exhale as you gently press the heel of your extended foot towards the floor.

- You should feel a stretch along the back of your calf muscle.

- Hold the stretch for several breaths, then release and repeat on the other side.

Benefits:

- Stretches the calf muscles, reducing tightness and improving flexibility in the lower legs.

- Alleviates discomfort associated with plantar fasciitis and Achilles tendonitis.

- Promotes better circulation and foot health.

Duration: Hold the seated calf stretch for 30-60 seconds on each leg, breathing deeply and allowing the muscles to relax.

19. Seated Pelvic Tilts

Steps:

- Sit comfortably on your chair with your feet flat on the floor and your hands resting on your thighs.

- Inhale deeply to lengthen your spine, then exhale as you tilt your pelvis forward, arching your lower back slightly.

- Hold the forward tilt for a few breaths, then inhale as you tilt your pelvis back, rounding your lower back and tucking your tailbone under.

- Continue to flow smoothly between forward and backward pelvic tilts, coordinating your breath with your movement.

Benefits:

- Improves mobility and flexibility in the hips and lower back.

- Strengthens the core muscles that support proper posture and alignment.

- Alleviates lower back pain and discomfort.

- Promotes awareness of pelvic alignment and body awareness.

Duration: Repeat the seated pelvic tilts for 5-10 breaths, moving slowly and mindfully with each tilt.

20. Seated Relaxation Pose

Steps:

- Sit comfortably on your chair with your feet flat on the floor and your hands resting on your thighs.

- Close your eyes and take several deep breaths, allowing your body to relax and soften with each exhale.

- Let go of any tension or tightness in your muscles, allowing them to melt into the support of the chair beneath you.

- Bring your awareness to your breath, observing the natural rhythm of inhalation and exhalation.

- Stay in this relaxed, meditative state for several minutes, allowing yourself to fully unwind and let go of any stress or worries.

Benefits:

- Promotes deep relaxation and stress relief.

- Reduces muscle tension and fatigue.

- Calms the mind and soothes the nervous system.

- Improves overall sense of well-being and inner peace.

Duration: Practice the seated relaxation pose for 5-10 minutes, or longer if desired, allowing yourself to sink into a state of deep relaxation and rejuvenation.

Chapter 4: Chair Yoga Cardio Exercises for Weight Loss

In this chapter, we'll explore different dynamic chair yoga exercises designed to elevate your heart rate, burn calories, and promote weight loss. These exercises are specifically tailored to provide a cardiovascular workout while remaining safe and accessible for seniors. Let's dive into each exercise:

1. Chair Jumping Jacks

Steps:

- Sit comfortably on your chair with your feet flat on the floor and your hands resting on your thighs.

- Inhale deeply, then exhale as you jump both feet out to the sides while simultaneously raising your arms overhead.

- Inhale as you jump your feet back together and lower your arms to your sides.

- Continue to perform jumping jacks at a steady pace, focusing on maintaining proper form and breathing rhythmically.

Benefits:

- Raises the heart rate and increases cardiovascular endurance.

- Engages multiple muscle groups, including the legs, arms, and core.

- Improves coordination and agility.

- Burns calories and promotes weight loss.

Duration: Perform chair jumping jacks for 1-2 minutes, gradually increasing the duration as your fitness level improves.

2. Seated High Knees

Steps:

- Sit tall on your chair with your feet flat on the floor and your hands resting on your thighs.

- Inhale deeply, then exhale as you lift one knee towards your chest, bringing it as high as you comfortably can.

- Lower the lifted leg back to the floor and repeat the movement with the opposite leg.

- Continue to alternate lifting your knees as quickly as possible while maintaining good posture and engaging your core muscles.

Benefits:

- Elevates the heart rate and boosts circulation.

- Targets the muscles of the lower body, including the quadriceps, hamstrings, and hip flexors.

- Improves balance and coordination.

- Burns calories and aids in weight loss.

Duration: Perform seated high knees for 1-2 minutes, gradually increasing the duration and intensity as you build endurance.

3. Seated Mountain Climbers

Steps:

- Sit tall on your chair with your feet flat on the floor and your hands resting on your thighs.

- Inhale deeply, then exhale as you lift one foot off the floor and drive your knee towards your chest.

- Quickly switch legs, bringing the opposite knee towards your chest while simultaneously lowering the other foot back to the floor.

- Continue to alternate between legs at a rapid pace, maintaining a steady rhythm and engaging your core muscles throughout the movement.

Benefits:

- Increases heart rate and cardiovascular fitness.

- Targets the core muscles, including the abdominals and obliques.

- Strengthens the muscles of the lower body, including the quadriceps, hamstrings, and calves.

- Enhances agility and coordination.

Duration: Perform seated mountain climbers for 1-2 minutes, gradually increasing the duration as your fitness level improves.

4. Chair Squat Jumps

Steps:

- Sit on the edge of your chair with your feet flat on the floor and your knees bent at a 90-degree angle.

- Inhale deeply, then exhale as you push through your heels to lift your hips off the chair and jump up into the air.

- Land softly on the balls of your feet, immediately lowering back down into a squat position with your hips hovering just above the chair.

- Repeat the squat jump motion, moving as quickly and explosively as you can while maintaining control and proper form.

Benefits:

- Raises the heart rate and boosts cardiovascular endurance.

- Targets the muscles of the lower body, including the quadriceps, glutes, and calves.

- Improves explosive power and strength.

- Burns calories and promotes weight loss.

Duration: Perform chair squat jumps for 1-2 minutes, taking breaks as needed to rest and recover between sets.

5. Seated Leg Swings

Steps:

1. Sit comfortably on your chair with your back straight and feet flat on the floor.

2. Hold onto the sides of the chair for support.

3. Extend one leg straight out in front of you, keeping it parallel to the floor.

4. Swing the extended leg gently forward and backward, focusing on the movement coming from the hip joint.

5. Perform the swinging motion for a set number of repetitions or time, then switch to the other leg.

Benefits:
- Loosens up the hip joints and improves hip mobility.

- Engages the muscles of the core and legs for stability.

- Helps improve balance and coordination.

- Can alleviate stiffness and discomfort in the hips.

Duration: Perform 10-15 swings on each leg, gradually increasing the number as you become more comfortable with the movement.

6. Seated Toe Taps

Steps:

1. Sit tall on your chair with your feet flat on the floor and your hands resting on your thighs.

2. Lift one foot off the floor and extend it forward, keeping the leg straight.

3. Tap the toes of the extended foot lightly on the floor in front of you.

4. Return the extended foot back to the starting position and repeat with the other leg.

5. Continue to alternate between legs, tapping the toes in a rhythmic motion.

Benefits:

- Targets the muscles of the lower body, including the quadriceps, hamstrings, and calves.

- Improves circulation in the legs and feet.

- Enhances flexibility in the ankles and toes.

- Can help alleviate stiffness and discomfort from prolonged sitting.

Duration: Perform 10-15 toe taps on each leg, gradually increasing the number as you become more comfortable with the movement.

7. Chair Step-Ups

Steps:

1. Stand in front of your chair with your feet hip-width apart and your hands on your hips.

2. Place one foot firmly on the seat of the chair, ensuring that it is stable and secure.

3. Press through the heel of the elevated foot to lift your body up onto the chair, straightening the leg fully.

4. Step back down to the floor with control, returning to the starting position.

5. Repeat the step-up motion with the same leg for a set number of repetitions, then switch to the other leg.

Benefits:

- Strengthens the muscles of the lower body, including the quadriceps, glutes, and calves.

- Improves balance and coordination.

- Provides a cardiovascular challenge when performed at a brisk pace.

- Can be modified to suit individual fitness levels by adjusting the height of the chair.

Duration: Perform 10-15 step-ups on each leg, gradually increasing the number as you become more comfortable with the movement.

8. Seated Arm Circles

Steps:

1. Sit tall on your chair with your feet flat on the floor and your hands resting on your thighs.

2. Extend your arms out to the sides at shoulder height, palms facing down.

3. Begin to make small circles with your arms, moving them forward in a controlled motion.

4. Continue to increase the size of the circles, gradually making them larger and more expansive.

5. After a set number of repetitions, reverse the direction of the circles and perform them in a backward motion.

Benefits:

- Mobilizes the shoulder joints and improves range of motion.

- Engages the muscles of the arms, shoulders, and upper back.

- Enhances circulation and blood flow to the upper body.

- Can help alleviate tension and stiffness in the shoulders and neck.

Duration: Perform 10-15 arm circles in each direction, gradually increasing the number and size of the circles as you become more comfortable with the movement.

9. Seated Punches

Steps:

1. Sit comfortably on your chair with your feet flat on the floor and your spine tall.

2. Bring your fists up to shoulder height, keeping your elbows bent and close to your sides.

3. Exhale as you extend one arm forward in a punching motion, rotating your palm down as you do so.

4. Inhale as you retract your arm back to the starting position, then repeat the motion with the opposite arm.

5. Continue to alternate punching arms at a steady pace, engaging your core muscles and maintaining good posture throughout the movement.

Benefits:

- Increases heart rate and boosts cardiovascular endurance.

- Targets the muscles of the arms, shoulders, and chest.

- Improves coordination and agility.

- Releases tension and stress in the upper body.

Duration: Perform seated punches for 1-2 minutes, gradually increasing the duration as your fitness level improves.

10. Seated Bicycle Crunches

Steps:

1. Sit tall on your chair with your feet flat on the floor and your hands lightly resting behind your head.

2. Lift your feet off the floor and bring your knees towards your chest, engaging your core muscles.

3. Inhale deeply, then exhale as you extend one leg out straight while simultaneously twisting your torso to bring the opposite elbow towards the bent knee.

4. Inhale to return to the starting position, then exhale as you switch sides, extending the opposite leg and twisting towards the other knee.

5. Continue to alternate between sides in a fluid, bicycle pedaling motion, focusing on keeping your core engaged and your movements controlled.

Benefits:

- Targets the muscles of the core, including the abdominals and obliques.

- Increases abdominal strength and definition.

- Improves flexibility and mobility in the spine.

- Enhances coordination and balance.

Duration: Perform seated bicycle crunches for 1-2 minutes, maintaining a steady pace and focusing on quality of movement over speed.

11. Seated Heel Taps

Steps:

1. Sit tall on your chair with your feet flat on the floor and your knees bent at a 90-degree angle.

2. Extend one leg out in front of you, keeping the foot flexed and the heel lifted off the floor.

3. Inhale deeply, then exhale as you reach towards the lifted heel with the opposite hand, tapping it lightly.

4. Inhale to return to the starting position, then exhale as you switch sides, tapping the other heel with the opposite hand.

5. Continue to alternate between sides in a controlled, rhythmic motion, engaging your core muscles and maintaining good posture throughout the movement.

Benefits:

- Targets the muscles of the core, including the abdominals and obliques.

- Improves coordination and balance.

- Increases flexibility and mobility in the hips and lower back.

- Helps to alleviate tightness and tension in the lower body.

Duration: Perform seated heel taps for 1-2 minutes, moving at a steady pace and focusing on maintaining proper form throughout the exercise.

12. Seated Side Leg Lifts

Steps:

1. Sit tall on your chair with your feet flat on the floor and your hands resting lightly on the sides of the chair for support.

2. Inhale deeply, then exhale as you lift one leg out to the side, keeping it straight and parallel to the floor.

3. Hold the lifted leg for a moment, engaging the muscles of the outer thigh and hip.

4. Inhale to lower the leg back down to the starting position, then exhale as you repeat the movement on the opposite side.

5. Continue to alternate between legs in a controlled, fluid motion, focusing on maintaining stability and balance throughout the exercise.

Benefits:

- Targets the muscles of the outer thighs, hips, and glutes.

- Improves hip stability and mobility.

- Enhances balance and coordination.

- Helps to prevent and alleviate hip and knee pain.

Duration: Perform seated side leg lifts for 1-2 minutes on each leg, maintaining a steady pace and focusing on quality of movement.

13. Seated Torso Twists

Steps:

1. Sit tall on your chair with your feet flat on the floor and your hands resting on your thighs.

2. Inhale deeply to lengthen your spine, then exhale as you twist your torso to the right, bringing your left hand to the outside of your right thigh and your right hand to the back of the chair.

3. Hold the twist for a few breaths, feeling a gentle stretch along the spine and through the torso.

4. Inhale to return to center, then exhale as you twist your torso to the left, bringing your right hand to the outside of your left thigh and your left hand to the back of the chair.

5. Hold the twist for a few breaths, then return to center and repeat on the other side.

Benefits:

- Improves spinal mobility and flexibility.

- Stretches the muscles of the spine, abdomen, and obliques.

- Stimulates digestion and detoxification.

- Promotes relaxation and relieves tension in the back and shoulders.

Duration: Hold each seated torso twist for 5-10 breaths on each side, moving slowly and mindfully with each twist.

14. Seated Jumping Jacks with Resistance Band

Steps:

1. Sit tall on your chair with your feet flat on the floor and your spine straight.

2. Place a resistance band around your thighs, just above the knees, and hold onto the ends of the band with your hands.

3. Inhale deeply, then exhale as you press against the resistance band to jump both feet out to the sides.

4. Inhale to return to the starting position, then exhale as you jump your feet back together.

5. Continue to perform seated jumping jacks at a steady pace, engaging your core muscles and pressing against the resistance band with each movement.

Benefits:

- Increases heart rate and boosts cardiovascular endurance.

- Strengthens the muscles of the legs, hips, and core.

- Improves coordination and agility.

- Burns calories and promotes weight loss.

Duration: Perform seated jumping jacks with resistance band for 1-2 minutes, gradually increasing the duration as your fitness level improves.

15. Seated Knee Lifts with Resistance Band

Steps:

1. Sit tall on your chair with your feet flat on the floor and your spine straight.

2. Place a resistance band around your thighs, just above the knees, and hold onto the ends of the band with your hands.

3. Inhale deeply, then exhale as you lift one knee towards your chest, pressing against the resistance band with the opposite leg.

4. Lower the lifted leg back to the floor, then repeat the movement with the opposite leg.

5. Continue to alternate lifting your knees at a steady pace, engaging your core muscles and pressing against the resistance band with each movement.

Benefits:

- Targets the muscles of the legs, hips, and core.

- Increases heart rate and boosts circulation.

- Improves balance and stability.

- Burns calories and promotes weight loss.

Duration: Perform seated knee lifts with resistance band for 1-2 minutes, alternating between legs with each repetition.

16. Seated Cross Punches

Steps:

1. Sit tall on your chair with your feet flat on the floor and your hands in loose fists by your sides.

2. Inhale deeply, then exhale as you twist your torso to the right, extending your left arm across your body in a punching motion.

3. Inhale to return to center, then exhale as you twist your torso to the left, extending your right arm across your body in a punching motion.

4. Continue to alternate between twisting and punching at a steady pace, engaging your core muscles and keeping your movements controlled and deliberate.

Benefits:

- Targets the muscles of the arms, shoulders, and core.

- Increases heart rate and boosts cardiovascular endurance.

- Improves coordination and agility.

- Burns calories and promotes weight loss.

Duration: Perform seated cross punches for 1-2 minutes, maintaining a steady rhythm and focusing on proper form with each punch.

17. Seated Torso Circles

Steps:

1. Sit comfortably on your chair with your feet flat on the floor and your hands resting on your thighs.

2. Inhale deeply and lengthen your spine, sitting tall with your shoulders relaxed.

3. Exhale as you gently rotate your torso to the right, bringing your right shoulder towards your right hip.

4. Inhale as you come back to center, then exhale as you rotate your torso to the left, bringing your left shoulder towards your left hip.

5. Continue to flow smoothly between right and left torso rotations, coordinating your breath with your movement.

6. Focus on creating a gentle circular motion with your torso, moving with awareness and control.

Benefits:

- Improves spinal mobility and flexibility.

- Releases tension and tightness in the back and waist.

- Stimulates digestion and massages the internal organs.

- Promotes relaxation and stress relief.

Duration: Perform seated torso circles for 1-2 minutes, alternating between clockwise and counterclockwise rotations.

18. Seated Jogging in Place

Steps:

1. Sit tall on your chair with your feet flat on the floor and your hands resting on your thighs.

2. Begin by lifting one foot off the floor and gently bouncing on the ball of that foot, mimicking a jogging motion.

3. As you lift one foot, simultaneously lift the opposite arm, bending your elbow and bringing your hand towards your shoulder.

4. Continue to alternate between lifting your feet and pumping your arms, moving at a pace that challenges you but allows you to maintain good form.

5. Focus on keeping your core engaged and your upper body tall and stable throughout the movement.

Benefits:

- Increases heart rate and cardiovascular endurance.

- Improves circulation and boosts energy levels.

- Engages the muscles of the legs, arms, and core.

- Burns calories and aids in weight loss.

Duration: Perform seated jogging in place for 1-2 minutes, gradually increasing the intensity and speed as your fitness level improves.

19. Seated Cross Body Reaches

Steps:

1. Sit tall on your chair with your feet flat on the floor and your hands resting on your thighs.

2. Inhale deeply, then exhale as you reach your right hand across your body towards your left knee, twisting your torso slightly to the left.

3. Inhale as you come back to center, then exhale as you reach your left hand across your body towards your right knee, twisting your torso slightly to the right.

4. Continue to flow smoothly between right and left cross body reaches, moving with control and awareness.

5. Focus on lengthening through the spine and engaging your core muscles to support the twisting motion.

Benefits:

- Stretches the muscles along the sides of the torso and waist.

- Engages the obliques and core muscles.

- Improves spinal mobility and flexibility.

- Promotes balance and coordination.

Duration: Perform seated cross body reaches for 1-2 minutes, alternating between right and left reaches with each breath.

20. Seated Leg Extensions with Resistance Band

Steps:

1. Sit tall on your chair with your feet flat on the floor and your hands resting on your thighs.

2. Place a resistance band around the bottom of one foot, holding the ends of the band securely in your hands.

3. Inhale deeply, then exhale as you extend the banded leg straight out in front of you, flexing your foot and engaging your quadriceps.

4. Inhale as you bend the knee and return to the starting position, keeping tension on the resistance band throughout the movement.

5. Repeat the leg extension motion for several repetitions, then switch to the opposite leg.

6. Focus on maintaining good posture and control throughout the exercise, avoiding any jerky or uncontrolled movements.

Benefits:

- Strengthens the muscles of the legs, including the quadriceps and hamstrings.

- Improves knee stability and joint health.

- Enhances lower body strength and endurance.

- Provides resistance training to complement cardiovascular exercise.

Incorporate these seated chair yoga exercises into your daily routine to increase strength, flexibility, and cardiovascular fitness. Remember to listen to your body and modify the exercises as needed to suit your individual needs and abilities. With consistent practice, you'll experience the numerous benefits of chair yoga for seniors.

Chapter 5: Chair Yoga Routines in Under 10 Minutes

Here, we'll explore chair yoga routines that can be completed in under 10 minutes, perfect for busy days when you need a quick and effective practice to rejuvenate your body and mind. Each routine incorporates a combination of gentle stretches, strengthening poses, and mindful breathing exercises to leave you feeling refreshed and energized. Let's dive into the routines:

1. Seated Sun Salutation

Routine:

1. Sit tall on your chair with your feet flat on the floor and your hands resting on your thighs.

2. Inhale as you sweep your arms overhead, stretching tall towards the sky.

3. Exhale as you hinge forward from your hips, reaching your hands towards your feet or the floor.

4. Inhale as you lengthen your spine and lift your chest forward.

5. Exhale as you fold deeper into the stretch, relaxing your head and neck.

6. Inhale to slowly roll back up to a seated position, stacking each vertebra one at a time.

7. Repeat the seated sun salutation sequence for 3-5 rounds, moving with your breath and focusing on smooth, controlled movements.

Benefits:

- Increases flexibility and mobility in the spine and hamstrings.

- Opens up the chest and improves lung capacity.

- Stimulates circulation and boosts energy levels.

- Promotes a sense of grounding and presence.

Duration: Complete the seated sun salutation routine in 3-5 minutes, allowing for a few breaths in each position.

2. Seated Warrior Sequence

Routine:

1. Sit tall on your chair with your feet flat on the floor and your hands resting on your thighs.

2. Inhale as you reach your arms out to the sides, lifting them up towards the sky.

3. Exhale as you twist your torso to the right, bringing your left hand to your right knee and your right hand behind you on the chair.

4. Inhale as you lengthen through your spine, then exhale as you deepen the twist, gazing over your right shoulder.

5. Hold the twist for a few breaths, then inhale to come back to center and repeat on the opposite side.

6. Continue to flow smoothly between right and left twists, moving with your breath and maintaining good posture throughout the sequence.

Benefits:

- Stretches the muscles along the sides of the torso and waist.

- Strengthens the core muscles and improves stability.

- Enhances balance and coordination.

- Promotes mental focus and clarity.

Duration: Complete the seated warrior sequence in 2-3 minutes, spending several breaths in each twist.

3. Seated Tree Pose

Routine:

1. Sit tall on your chair with your feet flat on the floor and your hands resting on your thighs.

2. Inhale as you lift your right foot off the floor, placing the sole of your right foot on the inside of your left thigh.

3. Exhale as you press your right foot firmly into your left thigh, rooting down through your sitting bones.

4. Inhale to lengthen through your spine, reaching your arms overhead.

5. Exhale as you bring your hands together in front of your heart in a prayer position.

6. Hold the seated tree pose for a few breaths, then release and repeat on the opposite side.

Benefits:

- Improves balance and stability.

- Strengthens the muscles of the legs and core.

- Opens up the hips and stretches the inner thighs.

- Cultivates focus and concentration.

Duration: Hold the seated tree pose for 1-2 minutes on each side, focusing on steady breathing and a stable foundation.

4. Seated Eagle Arms

Routine:

1. Sit tall on your chair with your feet flat on the floor and your hands resting on your thighs.

2. Inhale as you sweep your arms out to the sides, reaching them up towards the sky.

3. Exhale as you cross your right arm over your left arm, bringing the backs of your hands together or clasping your palms if possible.

4. Inhale to lift your elbows slightly, creating space between your shoulder blades.

5. Exhale as you lower your chin towards your chest, rounding your upper back slightly.

6. Hold the seated eagle arms stretch for a few breaths, then release and repeat with the opposite arm on top.

Benefits:

- Stretches the muscles of the shoulders, upper back, and arms.

- Improves posture and relieves tension in the neck and shoulders.

- Enhances circulation and blood flow.

- Encourages a sense of release and surrender.

Duration: Hold the seated eagle arms stretch for 1-2 minutes, focusing on deep, steady breathing and maintaining alignment.

5. Seated Chair Pose

Steps:

1. Sit tall on your chair with your feet flat on the floor and your hands resting on your thighs.

2. Inhale deeply and lengthen your spine, lifting your chest towards the sky.

3. Exhale as you bend your knees and lower your hips towards the edge of the chair, as if you were sitting back in an imaginary chair.

4. Keep your knees stacked directly over your ankles and your thighs parallel to the floor.

5. Reach your arms overhead, palms facing each other or coming together in prayer position.

6. Hold the seated chair pose for several breaths, feeling the strength and stability in your legs and core.

7. To come out of the pose, inhale as you straighten your legs and return to a seated position.

Benefits:

- Strengthens the muscles of the legs, including the quadriceps, hamstrings, and glutes.

- Improves balance and stability.

- Engages the core muscles and supports proper posture.

- Stimulates circulation and energy flow throughout the body.

Duration: Hold the seated chair pose for 30-60 seconds, gradually increasing the duration as you build strength and endurance.

6. Seated Forward Bend with Twist

Steps:

1. Sit tall on your chair with your feet flat on the floor and your hands resting on your thighs.

2. Inhale deeply and lengthen your spine, sitting tall with your shoulders relaxed.

3. Exhale as you hinge forward from your hips, reaching your hands towards your feet or the floor.

4. Inhale as you lengthen your spine even more, then exhale as you twist your torso to the right, placing your left hand on the outside of your right thigh.

5. Keep your right hand on the floor or reach it towards the back of the chair for support.

6. Hold the seated forward bend with twist for several breaths, feeling a deep stretch along the back of your legs and spine.

7. Inhale to come back to center, then exhale as you twist to the left, repeating the stretch on the opposite side.

Benefits:

- Stretches the muscles of the spine, hamstrings, and hips.

- Relieves tension in the back and shoulders.

- Massages the internal organs and aids in digestion.

- Increases spinal mobility and flexibility.

Duration: Hold each side of the seated forward bend with twist for 30-60 seconds, breathing deeply and surrendering to the stretch.

7. Seated Side Bend

Steps:

1. Sit tall on your chair with your feet flat on the floor and your hands resting on your thighs.

2. Inhale deeply and lengthen your spine, sitting tall with your shoulders relaxed.

3. Exhale as you reach your right arm overhead, stretching tall towards the sky.

4. Inhale to lengthen through your spine even more, then exhale as you lean to the left, creating a deep stretch along the right side of your body.

5. Keep both sitting bones rooted firmly on the chair and avoid collapsing into the stretch.

6. Hold the seated side bend for several breaths, feeling a gentle opening and lengthening along the right side of your torso.

7. Inhale to come back to center, then repeat the stretch on the opposite side.

Benefits:

- Stretches the muscles along the sides of the torso and waist.

- Increases flexibility and mobility in the spine.

- Opens up the chest and improves lung capacity.

- Promotes a sense of expansion and freedom in the body.

Duration: Hold each side of the seated side bend for 30-60 seconds, breathing deeply and sinking deeper into the stretch with each exhale.

8. Seated Cobra Pose

Steps:

1. Sit tall on your chair with your feet flat on the floor and your hands resting on your thighs.

2. Inhale deeply and lengthen your spine, lifting your chest towards the sky.

3. Exhale as you slide your hands down the sides of your legs, bringing your palms to rest on the tops of your thighs.

4. Inhale to draw your shoulder blades together and lift your chest even higher, arching your upper back.

5. Keep your shoulders relaxed and your neck long, avoiding any tension or strain.

6. Hold the seated cobra pose for several breaths, feeling a gentle stretch along the front of your torso and opening through your heart center.

7. Exhale to release the pose and come back to a neutral seated position.

Benefits:

- Opens up the chest and lungs, improving respiratory function.

- Strengthens the muscles of the back, including the erector spinae and rhomboids.

- Improves posture and alleviates tension in the shoulders and upper back.

- Stimulates digestion and massages the abdominal organs.

Duration: Hold the seated cobra pose for 30-60 seconds, breathing deeply and lifting your heart towards the sky with each inhale.

9. Seated Bridge Pose

Steps:

1. Sit comfortably on your chair with your feet flat on the floor and your hands resting on your thighs.

2. Inhale deeply and lengthen your spine, engaging your core muscles.

3. Exhale as you press firmly into your feet and lift your hips off the chair, coming into a bridge position.

4. Keep your knees aligned with your ankles and your thighs parallel to the floor.

5. Inhale as you hold the bridge pose, lifting your chest towards the ceiling and opening through the front of your body.

6. Exhale as you slowly lower your hips back down to the chair, returning to the starting position.

7. Repeat the seated bridge pose for several rounds, moving with your breath and focusing on the engagement of your core and leg muscles.

Benefits:

- Strengthens the muscles of the lower body, including the glutes, hamstrings, and quadriceps.

- Improves stability and balance.

- Stretches the spine and opens up the chest and shoulders.

- Stimulates circulation and boosts energy levels.

Duration: Hold the seated bridge pose for 3-5 breaths, repeating for 3-5 rounds.

10. Seated Meditation

Steps:

1. Sit comfortably on your chair with your feet flat on the floor and your hands resting on your thighs.

2. Close your eyes and take several deep breaths, allowing your body to relax and settle into the support of the chair.

3. Bring your awareness to your breath, observing the natural rhythm of inhalation and exhalation.

4. Notice the sensations of the breath as it enters and leaves your body, feeling the rise and fall of your chest and belly.

5. Allow your mind to become quiet and still, letting go of any thoughts or distractions that arise.

6. If your mind starts to wander, gently bring your focus back to the sensation of the breath, using it as an anchor to keep you present in the moment.

7. Continue to sit in meditation for as long as feels comfortable, allowing yourself to experience a sense of peace and tranquility.

Benefits:

- Reduces stress and anxiety.

- Improves focus and concentration.

- Cultivates mindfulness and self-awareness.

- Promotes emotional well-being and inner peace.

Duration: Practice seated meditation for 5-10 minutes or longer, depending on your preference and availability.

11. Seated Cat-Cow Flow

Steps:

1. Sit comfortably on your chair with your feet flat on the floor and your hands resting on your thighs.

2. Inhale as you arch your spine, lifting your chest and tilting your pelvis forward (Cow Pose).

3. Exhale as you round your spine, tucking your chin to your chest and drawing your belly button towards your spine (Cat Pose).

4. Continue to flow smoothly between Cat and Cow Poses, coordinating your breath with your movement.

5. Allow the movement to be gentle and fluid, focusing on creating space and flexibility in the spine.

6. Repeat the Cat-Cow flow for several rounds, moving with your breath and listening to your body's cues.

Benefits:

- Improves spinal flexibility and mobility.

- Releases tension in the back, neck, and shoulders.

- Massages the internal organs and stimulates digestion.

- Promotes relaxation and stress relief.

Duration: Flow through seated Cat-Cow poses for 3-5 minutes, moving at a pace that feels comfortable and sustainable.

12. Seated Warrior II Flow

Steps:

1. Sit tall on your chair with your feet flat on the floor and your hands resting on your thighs.

2. Inhale as you sweep your arms out to the sides, reaching them up towards the sky.

3. Exhale as you bend your right elbow and bring your right hand behind your head, reaching your left hand down towards the floor.

4. Inhale to lengthen through your spine, then exhale as you lean your upper body towards the right, creating a side stretch along your left side.

5. Hold the seated side stretch for a few breaths, then inhale to come back to center and repeat on the opposite side.

6. Continue to flow smoothly between right and left side stretches, moving with your breath and maintaining good posture throughout the sequence.

Benefits:

- Stretches the muscles along the sides of the torso and waist.

- Opens up the chest and improves lung capacity.

- Increases flexibility in the spine and shoulders.

- Promotes balance and stability.

Duration: Complete the seated Warrior II flow for 3-5 minutes, alternating between right and left side stretches with each breath.

13. Seated Balance Flow

Routine:

1. Sit tall on your chair with your feet flat on the floor and your hands resting on your thighs.

2. Inhale deeply as you lift your right knee towards your chest, balancing on your left foot.

3. Exhale as you extend your right leg forward, flexing your foot and engaging your core.

4. Inhale to draw your right knee back towards your chest, then exhale to extend the leg straight out to the side.

5. Continue to flow smoothly between knee lifts and leg extensions, moving with your breath and maintaining a steady balance.

6. Repeat the sequence on the opposite side, lifting and extending the left leg.

Benefits:

- Improves balance and stability.

- Strengthens the muscles of the legs, core, and hips.

- Increases focus and concentration.

- Promotes a sense of grounding and presence.

Duration: Complete the seated balance flow for 3-5 minutes, alternating between right and left sides.

14. Seated Gentle Flow for Energy

Routine:

1. Sit tall on your chair with your feet flat on the floor and your hands resting on your thighs.

2. Inhale deeply as you sweep your arms overhead, stretching tall towards the sky.

3. Exhale as you hinge forward from your hips, reaching your hands towards your feet or the floor.

4. Inhale to lengthen your spine and lift your chest forward.

5. Exhale as you fold deeper into the stretch, relaxing your head and neck.

6. Inhale to slowly roll back up to a seated position, stacking each vertebra one at a time.

7. Repeat the forward fold sequence several times, moving with your breath and allowing the movement to flow smoothly.

7. Hold the twist for a few breaths, then inhale to come back to center and repeat on the opposite side.

8. Continue to flow smoothly between stretches, moving with your breath and allowing the movement to feel natural and effortless.

Benefits:

- Increases flexibility and mobility in the spine, shoulders, and hips.

- Relieves tension and tightness in the muscles.

- Improves posture and alignment.

- Promotes a sense of relaxation and well-being.

Duration: Complete the seated chair yoga stretch routine for 5-7 minutes, focusing on deep, mindful breathing and gentle movement.

16. Seated Core Strengthening Flow

Routine:

1. Sit tall on your chair with your feet flat on the floor and your hands resting on your thighs.

2. Inhale deeply as you engage your core muscles and lift your arms overhead, reaching tall towards the sky.

3. Exhale as you twist your torso to the right, bringing your left elbow towards your right knee.

4. Inhale to come back to center, then exhale to twist to the left, bringing your right elbow towards your left knee.

5. Continue to flow smoothly between right and left twists, moving with your breath and engaging your core with each movement.

6. After several rounds of twists, inhale as you extend your arms forward and lift your legs off the floor, balancing on your sitting bones.

7. Exhale as you lower your arms and legs back down to the starting position.

8. Repeat the core strengthening flow for several rounds, focusing on maintaining stability and control throughout the movements.

Benefits:

- Strengthens the muscles of the core, including the abdominals, obliques, and lower back.

- Improves stability and balance.

- Enhances posture and alignment.

- Increases awareness of core engagement and activation.

Duration: Complete the seated core strengthening flow for 3-5 minutes, focusing on quality of movement and engagement of the core muscles.

17. Seated Chair Yoga Relaxation Sequence

Routine:

1. Sit comfortably on your chair with your feet flat on the floor and your hands resting on your thighs.

2. Close your eyes and take several deep breaths, inhaling through your nose and exhaling through your mouth.

3. Inhale as you sweep your arms overhead, stretching tall towards the sky.

4. Exhale as you bring your hands down to rest on your lap, palms facing up.

5. Continue to breathe deeply and slowly, allowing each exhale to release tension and stress from your body.

6. With each breath, visualize yourself sinking deeper into relaxation, feeling calm and at ease.

7. Stay in this seated relaxation pose for several minutes, allowing yourself to fully unwind and let go.

Benefits:

- Promotes deep relaxation and stress relief.

- Calms the nervous system and reduces anxiety.

- Releases tension in the muscles and joints.

- Improves overall sense of well-being and inner peace.

Duration: Practice the seated chair yoga relaxation sequence for 5-10 minutes, or longer if desired, allowing yourself to fully surrender to the present moment.

18. Seated Chair Yoga Flow for Better Sleep

Routine:

1. Sit comfortably on your chair with your feet flat on the floor and your hands resting on your thighs.

2. Inhale deeply as you sweep your arms overhead, stretching tall towards the sky.

3. Exhale as you hinge forward from your hips, reaching your hands towards your feet or the floor.

4. Inhale to lengthen your spine and lift your chest forward.

5. Exhale as you fold deeper into the stretch, relaxing your head and neck.

6. Inhale to slowly roll back up to a seated position, stacking each vertebra one at a time.

7. Repeat the seated sun salutation sequence for 3-5 rounds, moving with your breath and focusing on smooth, controlled movements.

8. Finish with a few minutes of seated meditation or deep breathing to calm the mind and prepare for sleep.

Benefits:

- Relieves tension and stiffness in the muscles and joints.

- Calms the mind and reduces racing thoughts.

- Improves circulation and promotes relaxation.

- Prepares the body and mind for restful sleep.

Duration: Complete the seated chair yoga flow for better sleep in 5-7 minutes, moving slowly and mindfully with each breath.

19. Seated Chair Yoga for Stress Relief

Routine:

1. Sit comfortably on your chair with your feet flat on the floor and your hands resting on your thighs.

2. Close your eyes and take several deep breaths, inhaling deeply through your nose and exhaling fully through your mouth.

3. Inhale as you sweep your arms overhead, stretching tall towards the sky.

4. Exhale as you twist your torso to the right, bringing your left hand to your right knee and your right hand behind you on the chair.

5. Inhale to lengthen through your spine, then exhale as you deepen the twist, gazing over your right shoulder.

6. Hold the twist for a few breaths, then inhale to come back to center and repeat on the opposite side.

7. Continue to flow smoothly between right and left twists, moving with your breath and focusing on releasing tension with each exhale.

8. Finish with a few minutes of deep breathing or seated meditation to further calm the mind and promote relaxation.

Benefits:

- Relieves tension and tightness in the muscles and joints.

- Calms the nervous system and reduces stress hormones.

- Increases oxygen flow to the brain, promoting mental clarity and focus.

- Enhances overall sense of well-being and inner peace.

Duration: Practice the seated chair yoga for stress relief routine for 5-7 minutes, or longer if needed, allowing yourself to fully surrender to the present moment and let go of stress and worries.

20. Seated Chair Yoga for Better Posture

Routine:

1. Sit tall on your chair with your feet flat on the floor and your hands resting on your thighs.

2. Inhale deeply as you lengthen through your spine, lifting your chest towards the sky.

3. Exhale as you draw your shoulder blades down and back, engaging the muscles between your shoulder blades.

4. Inhale to lift your arms overhead, reaching towards the sky with your fingertips.

5. Exhale as you lower your arms back down to your sides, keeping your shoulders relaxed and your chest open.

6. Continue to flow smoothly between seated mountain pose and shoulder rolls, moving with your breath and focusing on maintaining good posture throughout the sequence.

7. Finish with a few minutes of seated meditation or deep breathing to integrate the benefits of the practice and reinforce good posture habits.

Benefits:

- Improves spinal alignment and reduces strain on the neck and back.

- Strengthens the muscles of the upper back and shoulders.

- Opens up the chest and improves lung capacity.

- Enhances confidence and self-esteem.

Duration: Complete the seated chair yoga for better posture routine in 5-7 minutes, moving mindfully and with awareness of your alignment.

Incorporate these seated chair yoga routines into your daily schedule to promote relaxation, better sleep, stress relief, and improved posture. Adjust the duration and intensity of each routine to suit your individual needs and preferences, and enjoy the transformative benefits of chair yoga wherever you are.

Chapter 6: Nutrition and Diet Tips for Senior Weight Loss

Eating well is a cornerstone of good health at any age, but it becomes increasingly important as we grow older, especially for seniors embarking on a weight loss journey. In this chapter, we'll delve into the significance of nutrition for senior health and weight loss, exploring the vital role that proper diet plays in achieving and maintaining a healthy weight as we age.

Importance of Nutrition for Senior Health and Weight Loss:

Nutrition serves as the foundation upon which our health is built, influencing everything from our energy levels and immune function to our cognitive abilities and overall well-being. For seniors, maintaining a balanced and nutritious diet is essential not only for managing weight but also for preventing chronic diseases, supporting muscle mass and bone density, and promoting longevity.

One of the primary challenges that seniors face when it comes to nutrition and weight management is the natural decline in metabolic rate and muscle mass that occurs with aging. As we age, our bodies become less efficient at burning calories and metabolizing nutrients, making it easier to gain weight and harder to lose it. Additionally, factors such as changes in taste and smell, dental issues, medication side effects, and decreased appetite can further complicate dietary intake for seniors.

However, despite these challenges, prioritizing nutrient-dense foods and adopting healthy eating habits can significantly improve senior health and aid in weight loss efforts. A balanced diet rich in fruits, vegetables, whole grains, lean proteins, and healthy fats provides the essential nutrients, vitamins, and minerals that seniors need to thrive. These nutrient-dense foods not only support overall health but also help seniors feel fuller for longer, reducing the likelihood of overeating and promoting weight loss.

In addition to focusing on nutrient quality, portion control and mindful eating are crucial components of senior weight loss. Seniors should aim to consume smaller, more frequent meals throughout the day to maintain steady energy levels and prevent overeating. Practicing mindful eating, which involves paying attention to hunger and fullness cues, savoring each bite, and avoiding distractions while eating, can help seniors become more attuned to their body's signals and make healthier food choices.

Furthermore, hydration plays a vital role in senior health and weight loss. Many seniors are at risk of dehydration due to age-related changes in thirst perception and kidney function, as well as certain medications that may increase urinary frequency. Adequate hydration is essential for supporting metabolism, digestion, and nutrient absorption, as well as regulating appetite and preventing overeating. Seniors should aim to drink plenty of water throughout the day and incorporate hydrating foods such as fruits, vegetables, and soups into their diet.

In conclusion, nutrition plays a fundamental role in senior health and weight loss, serving as the cornerstone of overall well-being and vitality. By prioritizing nutrient-dense foods, practicing portion control and mindful eating, and staying hydrated, seniors can support their weight loss goals while also improving their overall quality of life. It's never too late to adopt healthy eating habits and reap the benefits of a balanced diet, regardless of age.- Tips for Combining Chair Yoga with a Balanced Diet for Optimal Results

Chapter 7: Flexibility and Inflammation Reduction

In this chapter, we'll explore the importance of flexibility training for seniors and how it contributes to reducing inflammation in the body. Flexibility is a crucial component of overall health and well-being, particularly as we age, and incorporating regular flexibility exercises into our routine can have numerous benefits for senior health.

Benefits of Flexibility Training for Seniors:

1. **Improved Joint Health:** Flexibility exercises help to maintain and improve the range of motion in our joints, reducing

stiffness and enhancing mobility. For seniors, maintaining joint flexibility is essential for performing daily activities with ease and reducing the risk of falls and injuries.

2. Enhanced Muscle Function: Flexibility training helps to lengthen and stretch the muscles, promoting better muscle function and reducing the risk of muscle imbalances and injuries. By improving muscle flexibility, seniors can also alleviate tension and tightness in the muscles, leading to greater comfort and ease of movement.

3. Increased Circulation: Flexibility exercises stimulate blood flow to the muscles and tissues, promoting better circulation throughout the body. Improved circulation helps to deliver oxygen and nutrients to the cells, while also aiding in the removal of metabolic waste products and toxins. This can contribute to reduced inflammation and faster recovery from exercise and injury.

4. Better Posture and Alignment: Flexibility training helps to lengthen and align the muscles and connective tissues, supporting better posture and spinal alignment. For seniors, maintaining good posture is essential for reducing strain on the spine and supporting overall musculoskeletal health. By improving flexibility in key areas such as the hips, shoulders, and spine, seniors can reduce the risk of postural issues and associated pain.

5. Reduced Risk of Injury: Flexibility exercises help to improve the elasticity of the muscles and connective tissues, reducing the risk of strains, sprains, and other soft tissue injuries. By increasing the flexibility and resilience of the muscles and joints, seniors can move more freely and safely, both in their daily activities and during exercise.

6. Stress Relief and Relaxation: Flexibility training promotes relaxation and stress relief by encouraging deep breathing and mindful movement. Stretching exercises help to release tension and tightness in the muscles, leading to feelings of relaxation and well-being. For seniors, incorporating flexibility exercises into their routine can provide a calming and rejuvenating experience, helping to reduce stress and promote mental clarity.

7. Enhanced Functional Fitness: Flexibility training improves functional fitness by enhancing the ability to perform everyday tasks and activities with ease and efficiency. Seniors who maintain good flexibility are better able to bend, reach, and twist, making it easier to carry out tasks such as household chores, gardening, and recreational activities.

- Chair Yoga Poses to Improve Flexibility and Mobility:

Chair yoga offers a gentle yet effective way for seniors to improve flexibility and mobility, even for those with limited mobility or physical challenges. Here are some chair yoga poses specifically designed to enhance flexibility and mobility:

Benefits:

- Increases circulation and boosts energy levels.

- Stretches the muscles of the spine, hamstrings, and hips.

- Promotes relaxation and stress relief.

- Invigorates the body and mind.

Duration: Complete the seated gentle flow for energy for 3-5 minutes, moving with intention and mindfulness.

15. Seated Chair Yoga Stretch Routine

Routine:

1. Sit tall on your chair with your feet flat on the floor and your hands resting on your thighs.

2. Inhale deeply as you sweep your arms overhead, stretching tall towards the sky.

3. Exhale as you interlace your fingers and press your palms up towards the ceiling, lengthening through your spine.

4. Inhale to reach your arms out to the sides, opening up through the chest and shoulders.

5. Exhale as you twist your torso to the right, placing your left hand on your right knee and your right hand behind you on the chair.

6. Inhale to lengthen through your spine, then exhale to deepen the twist, gazing over your right shoulder.

1. Seated Forward Fold:

- Sit tall on the edge of your chair with your feet flat on the floor.

- Inhale to lengthen your spine, then exhale as you hinge forward from your hips, bringing your chest towards your thighs.

- Rest your hands on your shins, ankles, or the floor, depending on your flexibility.

- Hold the stretch for a few breaths, feeling a gentle stretch along the spine and the back of the legs.

- To come out of the pose, inhale as you slowly roll back up to a seated position.

2. Seated Spinal Twist:

- Sit tall on your chair with your feet flat on the floor and your hands resting on your thighs.

- Inhale to lengthen your spine, then exhale as you twist your torso to the right, bringing your left hand to the outside of your right knee and your right hand behind you on the chair.

- Hold the twist for a few breaths, feeling a gentle stretch along the spine and the muscles of the torso.

- Inhale to come back to center, then exhale as you repeat the twist on the opposite side.

- Continue to flow smoothly between right and left twists, moving with your breath.

3. Seated Cat-Cow Stretch:

- Sit tall on your chair with your feet flat on the floor and your hands resting on your thighs.

- Inhale as you arch your back and lift your chest towards the sky, bringing your shoulder blades together.

- Exhale as you round your spine and tuck your chin towards your chest, bringing your navel towards your spine.

- Continue to flow smoothly between cat and cow poses, moving with your breath and focusing on lengthening and mobilizing the spine.

4. Seated Shoulder Opener:

- Sit tall on your chair with your feet flat on the floor and your hands resting on your thighs.

- Inhale as you reach your arms out to the sides, lifting them up towards the sky.

- Exhale as you bring your arms behind you, interlacing your fingers and pressing your palms together.

- Hold the stretch for a few breaths, feeling a gentle opening across the chest and shoulders.

- Release the arms and repeat the stretch as needed.

- Techniques for Reducing Inflammation and Joint Pain Through Chair Yoga:

Chair yoga can be a valuable tool for reducing inflammation and joint pain, offering gentle movements and stretches that help alleviate discomfort and promote healing. Here are some techniques to help reduce inflammation and joint pain through chair yoga:

1. Gentle Movement: Engage in gentle, fluid movements that help lubricate the joints and reduce stiffness. Incorporate movements such as wrist circles, ankle rolls, and neck stretches to promote mobility and reduce inflammation in key areas.

2. Deep Breathing: Practice deep, diaphragmatic breathing to help calm the nervous system and reduce stress, which can exacerbate inflammation and pain. Focus on inhaling deeply through the nose and exhaling fully through the mouth, allowing each breath to be slow, smooth, and deliberate.

3. Mindfulness Meditation: Incorporate mindfulness meditation techniques to cultivate awareness of sensations in the body and promote relaxation. Focus on observing any areas of tension or discomfort without judgment, allowing them to soften and release with each breath.

4. Joint-Friendly Poses: Choose chair yoga poses that are gentle on the joints and promote flexibility without causing strain or discomfort. Poses such as seated mountain pose, gentle twists, and supported backbends can help improve circulation, reduce inflammation, and alleviate joint pain.

5. Relaxation Techniques: Dedicate time at the end of your chair yoga practice to relaxation techniques such as guided imagery, progressive muscle relaxation, or body scanning. These techniques can help reduce stress and tension throughout the body, leading to decreased inflammation and improved overall well-being.

By incorporating these chair yoga poses and techniques into your daily routine, you can effectively reduce inflammation and joint pain while promoting flexibility, mobility, and overall health and well-being. Remember to listen to your body and modify poses as needed to suit your individual needs and abilities. With consistent practice, you'll experience the transformative benefits of chair yoga on your inflammatory and joint health.

Chapter 8: Conclusion and Next Steps

As we conclude our journey through chair yoga for senior weight loss, let's take a moment to reflect on the key chair yoga poses and exercises that we've explored to support your wellness goals.

Recap of Key Chair Yoga Poses and Exercises for Senior Weight Loss:

1. Seated Cat-Cow Stretch: A gentle spinal mobility exercise that improves flexibility and reduces tension in the back and neck.

2. Seated Forward Fold: Helps lengthen the spine and hamstrings, promoting flexibility and relieving lower back discomfort.

3. Seated Spinal Twist: Enhances spinal mobility and stimulates digestion while releasing tension in the torso and back muscles.

4. Seated Mountain Pose: Promotes good posture and strengthens the core muscles, supporting overall stability and balance.

5. Chair Jumping Jacks: Increases heart rate and boosts cardiovascular fitness, aiding in weight loss and improving endurance.

6. Seated High Knees: Engages the leg muscles and elevates the heart rate, contributing to calorie burning and metabolic health.

7. Seated Torso Circles: Improves spinal flexibility and mobility while releasing tension in the back and waist.

8. Seated Jogging in Place: Boosts circulation and energy levels, supporting weight loss and overall cardiovascular health.

9. Seated Cross Body Reaches: Stretches the side body and improves range of motion, promoting better posture and flexibility.

10. Seated Leg Extensions with Resistance Band: Strengthens the leg muscles and supports joint health, enhancing mobility and stability.

These chair yoga poses and exercises are just a starting point on your journey to improved health and well-being. Remember that consistency and dedication are key to achieving your goals, and it's important to listen to your body and progress at your own pace.

As you continue your chair yoga practice, consider incorporating other healthy lifestyle habits such as mindful eating, staying hydrated, and getting regular exercise outside of your yoga practice. By taking a holistic approach to your wellness, you'll not only support your weight loss goals but also enhance your overall quality of life.

In closing, I encourage you to stay committed to your wellness journey and celebrate your progress along the way. Whether you're seeking to lose weight, improve flexibility, or simply enhance your overall health, chair yoga offers a safe, accessible, and effective way to support your goals and live your best life.

Encouragement for Continued Practice and Progress:

As you embark on your journey of chair yoga for senior weight loss, I want to offer you words of encouragement and support for your continued practice and progress.

First and foremost, I commend you for taking the initiative to prioritize your health and well-being. Making the decision to incorporate chair yoga into your daily routine is a powerful step towards achieving your wellness goals, and I applaud your commitment to self-care.

Remember that progress is not always linear, and it's normal to encounter challenges along the way. Whether you're struggling with consistency, facing physical limitations, or feeling discouraged by slow progress, know that every effort you make towards your health matters. Each time you show up on your mat, you are investing in your physical, mental, and emotional well-being, and that is something to be proud of.

Be gentle with yourself and practice self-compassion as you navigate your wellness journey. Celebrate even the smallest victories and milestones, whether it's holding a pose for an extra breath or noticing increased flexibility and strength over time. Every step forward, no matter how small, is a testament to your resilience and dedication.

When faced with challenges or setbacks, remember why you started this journey in the first place. Connect with your intrinsic motivation and remind yourself of the benefits you hope to gain from your practice. Whether it's improving your overall health, increasing mobility, or simply finding moments of peace and relaxation, hold onto these aspirations as sources of inspiration and motivation.

Surround yourself with a supportive community of fellow yogis, friends, and loved ones who uplift and encourage you on your path. Share your experiences, challenges, and successes with others who understand and empathize with your journey. Together, you can provide each other with strength, encouragement, and accountability as you navigate the ups and downs of your practice.

Lastly, trust in the process and have faith in your ability to create positive change in your life. Embrace the journey with an open heart and a curious mind, and allow yourself to be present in each moment of your practice. As you continue to show up for yourself with dedication and perseverance, you will undoubtedly experience growth, transformation, and a deepening sense of well-being.

You are capable, you are resilient, and you are worthy of investing in your health and happiness. Keep shining bright on your path of chair yoga for senior weight loss, and know that I am cheering you on every step of the way.

- Resources for Further Exploration and Support on the Senior Weight Loss Journey:

Embarking on a senior weight loss journey can be both empowering and challenging, but you don't have to go it alone. Here are some valuable resources to further explore and support you on your path to wellness:

1. Books on Senior Nutrition and Wellness: Dive deeper into the topics of nutrition, fitness, and holistic wellness with books written specifically for seniors. Look for titles that offer practical advice, evidence-based strategies, and inspirational stories to guide and motivate you on your journey.

2. Online Communities and Forums: Connect with like-minded individuals who are also navigating the senior weight loss journey by joining online communities and forums dedicated to health and wellness. These virtual spaces provide a supportive environment where you can share experiences, ask questions, and find encouragement from others who understand your challenges and goals.

3. Nutrition and Fitness Apps: Take advantage of technology to track your food intake, monitor your physical activity, and stay motivated on your weight loss journey. There are many apps available that cater specifically to seniors, offering customized meal plans, workout routines, progress tracking tools, and motivational resources to help you stay on track and achieve your goals.

4. Senior-Friendly Exercise Classes: Explore local community centers, gyms, and senior centers for exercise classes tailored to older adults. Look for classes that focus on low-impact activities such as chair yoga, gentle stretching, water aerobics, and tai chi, which offer numerous health benefits and can be adapted to accommodate varying fitness levels and abilities.

5. Professional Guidance and Support: Consider seeking guidance from healthcare professionals such as registered dietitians, certified personal trainers, and physical therapists who specialize in working with seniors. These professionals can provide personalized advice, create tailored nutrition and exercise plans, and offer ongoing support and encouragement to help you reach your weight loss goals safely and effectively.

6. Educational Workshops and Seminars: Attend workshops, seminars, and educational events focused on senior nutrition, fitness, and weight management. These events often feature expert speakers, interactive demonstrations, and practical tips to help you make informed decisions about your health and well-being.

7. Community Wellness Programs: Take advantage of community-based wellness programs and initiatives that offer resources, support, and activities for seniors looking to improve their health and fitness. These programs may include group exercise classes, nutrition workshops, health screenings, and social activities designed to promote overall well-being and foster a sense of community among participants.

By exploring these resources and tapping into the support and guidance available, you can enhance your senior weight loss journey and create a path to a healthier, happier, and more vibrant life. Remember that every step you take towards better health is a step in the right direction, and you deserve to prioritize your well-being and invest in yourself at every stage of life.

BONUS

Progress Tracker

Instructions:

1. Date: Begin by entering the date of your chair yoga session.

2. Session Duration: Record the duration of your chair yoga practice. Whether it's a quick 10-minute stretch or a more extended session, document the time spent.

3. Exercises Completed: Tick off the chair yoga exercises you completed during the session. Take note of any modifications or variations you explored.

4. Physical Feelings: Use this space to jot down how your body feels post-session. Pay attention to changes in flexibility, muscle tension, or any areas of improvement.

5. Mood and Energy: Describe your emotional state and energy levels before and after the session. Notice any positive shifts in mood or increased vitality.

6. General Notes: Share any observations or thoughts about your chair yoga practice. This could include challenges faced, breakthroughs experienced, or any modifications you found particularly beneficial.

WORKOUT LOG

	Activities	Tracker	Notes
MON		Session Duration: Exercises Completed: Physical Feelings	Date: Time: Mood and Energy:	

	Activities	Tracker	Notes
TUE		Session Duration: Exercises Completed: Physical Feelings	Date: Time: Mood and Energy:	

	Activities	Tracker	Notes
WED		Session Duration: Exercises Completed: Physical Feelings	Date: Time: Mood and Energy:	

	Activities	Tracker	Notes
THU		Session Duration: Exercises Completed: Physical Feelings	Date: Time: Mood and Energy:	

	Activities	Tracker	Notes
FRI		Session Duration: Exercises Completed: Physical Feelings	Date: Time: Mood and Energy:	

	Activities	Tracker	Notes
SAT		Session Duration: Exercises Completed: Physical Feelings	Date: Time: Mood and Energy:	

	Activities	Tracker	Notes
SUN		Session Duration: Exercises Completed: Physical Feelings	Date: Time: Mood and Energy:	

WORKOUT LOG

MON

Activities

Tracker

Session Duration:

Exercises Completed:

Physical Feelings

Date:

Time:

Mood and Energy:

Notes

TUE

Activities

Tracker

Session Duration:

Exercises Completed:

Physical Feelings

Date:

Time:

Mood and Energy:

Notes

WED

Activities

Tracker

Session Duration:

Exercises Completed:

Physical Feelings

Date:

Time:

Mood and Energy:

Notes

THU

Activities

Tracker

Session Duration:

Exercises Completed:

Physical Feelings

Date:

Time:

Mood and Energy:

Notes

FRI

Activities

Tracker

Session Duration:

Exercises Completed:

Physical Feelings

Date:

Time:

Mood and Energy:

Notes

SAT

Activities

Tracker

Session Duration:

Exercises Completed:

Physical Feelings

Date:

Time:

Mood and Energy:

Notes

SUN

Activities

Tracker

Session Duration:

Exercises Completed:

Physical Feelings

Date:

Time:

Mood and Energy:

Notes

WORKOUT LOG

	Activities	Tracker	Notes
MON		Session Duration: / Exercises Completed: / Physical Feelings	Date: / Time: / Mood and Energy:	
TUE		Session Duration: / Exercises Completed: / Physical Feelings	Date: / Time: / Mood and Energy:	
WED		Session Duration: / Exercises Completed: / Physical Feelings	Date: / Time: / Mood and Energy:	
THU		Session Duration: / Exercises Completed: / Physical Feelings	Date: / Time: / Mood and Energy:	
FRI		Session Duration: / Exercises Completed: / Physical Feelings	Date: / Time: / Mood and Energy:	
SAT		Session Duration: / Exercises Completed: / Physical Feelings	Date: / Time: / Mood and Energy:	
SUN		Session Duration: / Exercises Completed: / Physical Feelings	Date: / Time: / Mood and Energy:	

WEIGHT TRACKER

JANUARY

Week 1	Week 2	Week 3	Week 4
.lbs	.lbs	.lbs	.lbs

FEBRUARY

Week 1	Week 2	Week 3	Week 4
.lbs	.lbs	.lbs	.lbs

MARCH

Week 1	Week 2	Week 3	Week 4
.lbs	.lbs	.lbs	.lbs

Notes	Before	After
	.lbs	.lbs

TARGET WEIGHT

.lbs

WEIGHT TRACKER

APRIL

Week 1	Week 2	Week 3	Week 4
.lbs	.lbs	.lbs	.lbs

MAY

Week 1	Week 2	Week 3	Week 4
.lbs	.lbs	.lbs	.lbs

JUNE

Week 1	Week 2	Week 3	Week 4
.lbs	.lbs	.lbs	.lbs

Notes	Before	After
	.lbs	.lbs

TARGET WEIGHT

.lbs

WEIGHT TRACKER

JULY

Week 1	Week 2	Week 3	Week 4
.lbs	.lbs	.lbs	.lbs

AUGUST

Week 1	Week 2	Week 3	Week 4
.lbs	.lbs	.lbs	.lbs

SEPTEMBER

Week 1	Week 2	Week 3	Week 4
.lbs	.lbs	.lbs	.lbs

Notes	Before	After
	.lbs	.lbs

TARGET WEIGHT

.lbs

WEIGHT TRACKER

OCTOBER

Week 1	Week 2	Week 3	Week 4
.lbs	.lbs	.lbs	.lbs

NOVEMBER

Week 1	Week 2	Week 3	Week 4
.lbs	.lbs	.lbs	.lbs

DECEMBER

Week 1	Week 2	Week 3	Week 4
.lbs	.lbs	.lbs	.lbs

Notes	Before	After
	.lbs	.lbs

TARGET WEIGHT

.lbs

FOOD TRACKER

Date	Breakfast	Lunch	Dinner	Snack
SUN				
MON				
TUE				
WED				
THU				
FRI				
SAT				

Notes	Target Weight

FOOD TRACKER

Date	Breakfast	Lunch	Dinner	Snack
SUN				
MON				
TUE				
WED				
THU				
FRI				
SAT				

Notes	Target Weight

After reading and enjoying this book, you should consider getting a copy of its work.

Thanks for purchasing

Wishing you a fulfilling and transformative chair yoga journey!

Warm regards,

Eleanor Grace.

Send a mail to lareaderpublishing@gmail.com to claim your

Free audio book.

Scan to download our free audio book

Please do well to give a sincere reviews on amazon, and we're also open for corrections. Kindly drop your opinion in our email. Thanks for purchasing, God bless you.

www.ingramcontent.com/pod-product-compliance
Lightning Source LLC
Chambersburg PA
CBHW070811260726
48660CB00005B/1817